# How I Lost

# 50

# Pounds in

# 5

I0116308

# Seconds

## A Story of a New Life
## by Steve Fitzhugh

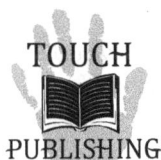

TOUCH
PUBLISHING

*How I Lost 50 Pounds in 5 Seconds*
Copyright © 2011, 2014 by Steve Fitzhugh

Published by:
Touch Publishing
P.O. Box 180303
Arlington, Texas 76096
www.TouchPublishingServices.com


Printed in the United States of America on acid-free paper

ISBN: 978-0-9937951-5-2
Library of Congress Control Number: 2014956360

Connect with Steve Fitzhugh: www.PowerMoves.org


Other books by Steve Fitzhugh:

*Pastor, We Need A Bigger Boat*
*The Adventures of Lil' Stevie*
*Who Will Survive?*
*Bringing the H.E.A.T.*

Find Steve's books through his website, online retailers, request them at your local bookstore, or through his publisher.

# Table of Contents

# Introduction

50/5

Five seconds! Imagine that. After years of failed weight loss attempts, I was able to lose half of my targeted weight reduction in only five seconds! It was no miracle diet, no expensive therapy, or radical infomercial that did the trick. In fact, there was almost zero dollars of added expense. I simply used a proven home remedy and five seconds later I was about 50 pounds lighter. In the chapters to follow I will share with you, in some detail, the four ingredients I applied beginning August 14th 2007. Then after September **2nd**, October **2nd**, November **2nd**, December **2nd**, and January **2nd** I had lost 46 pounds! That's almost 50 pounds in only five **seconds**!

Okay, okay I confess that was a play on words to get you to pick up this book, and it worked. I want people to read my short story because I can't believe how dramatically my whole life has changed by losing the excess weight. Life is more comfortable. I am much healthier and my quality of living has improved spectacularly. I went from a 44-inch waist to a 34-inch waist. My shirt size went from 3X down to a large. My suit jacket went from a size 52 to a 43 long. It wasn't easy, yet at the same time it wasn't that difficult. Consistency is all it took, along with some old school sweat equity. The discipline to make the tough decisions about what I put in my body, and how I exercise my body, was buoyed by what inspired me, and what I learned about health and life. As a friend once told me, "There is the pain of discipline and the pain of regret, either way there will be pain, so choose and be strong."

Cardiovascular disease, diabetes, and hypertension are completely preventable for 95% of people just by changing their diet and lifestyle. Hardened blood vessels kill more people worldwide than all of the other diseases combined and yet it is not only preventable in most cases, but reversible. Recent research has demonstrated the cessation of prostate tumor growth simply by making low-tech changes in diet and exercise. About 65% of adults and 15% of children are obese in America. At the same time diabetes has increased about 70% in 30 year olds in the last 10 years. These diseases are called lifestyle diseases because it's our lifestyle that contributes to their prevalence.

I changed my lifestyle so I can live. Everywhere I go people who have known me over the years are forced to take a second look when they see me since I have lost the weight. "Is Steve sick?" "Does he have AIDS?" "Is he on crack?" I have heard it all. I've even had people ask me to stop losing weight. One time I was told I was too thin. Ath that point I was at 220 pounds, well overweight for a 6-foot tall male. I did resume weight lifting to help my muscles recover from atrophy, but it's really not about anyone else's opinion, it's about a healthy lifestyle.

Darrell Green, NFL Hall of Famer and friend, once told me to find an exercise routine and make it the fabric of my lifestyle. One person said they felt safer around me when I was 280 pounds. I am not going to forfeit my health so someone else can feel safe! Most people applaud my weight loss and the fact that I have kept the weight off.

It's only been four years, but I've lost 93 pounds and I'm happy and healthy at a svelte 200 pounds, only 3 pounds heavier than my 1986 rookie year in the NFL. I've been asked so often how did I do it? I simply had to write my short story. This book is a mere snapshot of how and why I made lifestyle changes. There will never be an easier time to start than today. I can guarantee you, tomorrow will be more difficult. My hope is that you will be inspired to do the same thing that I did, beginning today, and pass the knowledge on.


Steve Fitzhugh
2011, Washington, DC

# Chapter 1

50/5

# "One Big Mac away from a massive stroke!"

It was August 14, 2007. I had just returned from a weeklong vacation in Scottsdale, Arizona. The week before, while on vacation I attempted some early morning jogging with my wife. It was embarrassing. At 6 a.m. it was already 90 degrees. I tried in earnest to keep up with my wife. She would talk to me throughout the run and at some point even ask questions. I would think to myself, "Why is she asking me something as if I have the breath to respond?" I was always too oxygen deprived to respond, or speak in general, whenever I attempted to run with my wife. I thought if I ran while on vacation I could impress my doctor at my physical check up the week we returned. It didn't work. I found myself just as fat, sitting today in the doctor's office. I can still hear Dr. Michalak's casual but very, very intentional words that he spoke to me that day.

"Steve," he said with mild exasperation in his foreign accent, "what we don't want is stroke."

He took another look at my blood sugar level, and re-read my blood pressure numbers, before slowly shaking his head in disapproval. For years he had been telling me, "Steve we must get pressure down. We must lose weight and exercise."

Hypertension–a.k.a. high blood pressure, the silent killer. I knew too well about its deadliness. My brother Raymond died from a massive hemorrhaging in his brain as a result of severe hypertension complicated by substance abuse. Knowing I was a former professional football player, Doc never felt he needed to go into detail about what it was going to take for me to get back in shape.

"Stephen, you played this American Football. You know what you must do. You know these things!"

Two years prior to this visit with Dr. Michalak,  he challenged me to get down to 240 pounds.

"Impossible!" I thought to myself.

Most of my adult life I was at least 270 pounds.  I have always been this big, thick diesel football player-looking dude. Most people excused my girth by surmising, "Steve's a football player, and they are supposed to be big." I had big thick arms, neck, legs, chest and head.  Most people didn't realize I played as a 197-pound free safety, 205 pounds at my heaviest in the NFL. As my girth grew, I used the 3X-Large, boxy "Fred Flintstone" shirts to become a master at hiding my fat midsection, my love handles, and my unsightly fat back. I always wore black because I thought it made me look thinner. That's like an elephant painting his toenails different colors so he can hide in the jellybean jar.

The first time Doc challenged me to lose weight I was 280 pounds. But at this visit, I was a hefty 293 pounds and Dr. Michalak went a step further. He went beyond his normal exhortations for me to be healthier.

Today he told me a story:

"I have brother-in-law, Stephen, in great health," he began (his English was stilted and broken and I'm writing it like he said it). "He runs every day, and is speaker like you." (This is where I became a little skeptical of this story because the main character was a speaker like me. Nevertheless, I respectfully continued listening.) "One day this young speaker, at merely 37 years, has massive stroke, all because he not take care of blood pressure. Today, to hear him speak you must practically put ear next to mouth. And when he walks he must walk like this..." The doc began to demonstrate by shuffling across the examination room slowly with his feet together traveling no more than an inch at a time with each step.

"This, Stephen, will be your fate without change. You will barely be able to speak; your words will be mostly mumble after stroke. After stroke it will take long time to just go across floor," he finished with a careful look into my eyes.

For the first time I associated my lack of discipline and consequent deteriorating health to the possible inability to support my family. There was silence in the room. This time, Dr. Michalak REALLY got my attention. In essence, my doctor had just told me I was one Big Mac away from a MASSIVE stroke.

I was 293 pounds and rarely, if ever, exercised. My blood pressure was 177 over 119. My blood sugar reading was well over 500. I had severe acid reflux. I snored horribly. I was chronically out of breath. I ate what I wanted, drank as much soda as I wanted, had as much dessert as I wanted and was killing myself at age 44 and didn't recognize it. People saw my smile on the outside but no one knew how miserable I was being severely overweight. Because of my work, I am frequently on airplanes and was always uncomfortable. Before taking my seat, I would extend the seatbelt to its limit so I wouldn't have to struggle to fasten it once I was seated. As a speaker, I had to request a towel for every presentation because shortly into my talk I was always covered with sweat. My niece once exclaimed when she saw me sweating, "Uncle Steve, you're raining!"

In between performing school assemblies I practically had to force myself to nap because I was so winded and exhausted. Even if it was only a 20-minute power nap in the car, I needed to rest. I was out of breath when I spoke and sang. On one occasion, in front of 3,000 people, I had to skip a line in a song because I couldn't breathe. Miserable. And what was worse is that I didn't know exactly how miserable I was. I was not just miserable, I was in essence killing myself. The day after my doctor visit, my wife was heading to the track complex for a run. As was her routine, she invited me to join her knowing I would say, "I'm too busy" or give some other lame excuse. I shocked her.

"Sure," I said.

"Whaattt?" she responded in surprise.

"I have a new motivation," I told her. "Mumble-mumble, shuffle-shuffle!"

This was the lasting impression Doc made on my life when he characterized what my motivational speaking would look like and sound like after my stroke. I explained that to my wife, and simply said, "I'm *not* going out like that!"

# Chapter 2

# How I Did It

50/5

How often does America try a new fad to lose weight? How often do we make New Years resolutions to finally rid ourselves of unsightly and unhealthy fat? Most of us relinquish those resolutions after only two months. I fell into this vicious cycle of pledges and promises and eventual disappointment. I had many failed attempts to lose the weight. My vows never lasted and the weight loss was never sustained. The difference for me this time was the combination of four elements.

Over a period of 15 years I made many attempts to regain my health by diet and exercise. My weight has fluctuated from 280 pounds to 270 to 275 to 290 and back to 280 pounds. When I hit 293 pounds I knew what had to be done, I just hadn't done it! Four elements/ingredients became what I like to call "lifesaver friends" of mine: Diet, Exercise, Education, and Motivation. Up to that point, diet and exercise were what I knew about. The real dynamite this time was education and the lit fuse was motivation.

I had to make a radical dietary lifestyle change if I wanted to live life to the fullest. I became brutally honest with myself. I kept it simple. Over the years I developed a modest knowledge of the good stuff to eat and the bad stuff to avoid. Flipping through the channels of late night television, you will learn about diet fads, strategies, sugars, and carbohydrates. I decided to go low carb and eliminate the sugar. Sweets, potatoes, pasta and bread were banned from my meal table. I went cold turkey for the first six weeks. I was serious. No sweets, cakes, cookies, sweet drinks, sodas, candies, or refined sugar of any kind. No sweet teas, raspberry teas, sugar in my coffee, no caramel macchiatos from Starbucks, chocolate chip cookies, or Chick-fil-A milkshakes.

*"Sugar equals poison,"* I said to myself time after time. I quickly lost 20 pounds. Losing the first twenty was great motivation. I had no idea how these menu items dominated my daily intake until I eliminated them. I mean, there were days that I would stop at 7-Eleven on my way home from work for my favorite: yellow Hostess cupcakes and Nestlé's strawberry milk. NO MORE! When analyzing your intake, you must be honest with yourself because it means life and death. Ask yourself: *What's my secret binge?* Personally, I would sit in the 7-Eleven parking lot eating my pastries so as not to have to explain the junk food wrappers in my truck to my wife. I thought: *"If I quickly eat in my truck, and if I stay in the parking lot, I can discard the hard evidence before ever reaching home. No one but me would know that I just pigged out on a sweet binge."*

In the past I made some of these same changes but I was uninformed about why these changes were important. Without the proper information, my changes had no foundation, only good intentions. With no real foundation or understanding for my changes, the change stopped and I returned to my bad habits after only a few weeks. With regards to my diet, it was through the education from my research that I began to understand how sweets worked in my life, in particular sugar.

I learned that my body only needs about 22-34 grams of sugar a day or in everyday terms, 4-6 teaspoons. Since I loved a big cup of Coke at my favorite fast food joint, I went to the Coke website to see exactly how many grams of sugar were contained in one medium sized (16 ounces) bottle. Much to my surprise, the people at Coke do not list sugar as an ingredient in its Coke product. I flipped through to their Dasani water page and sure enough I saw sugar listed as an ingredient and the amount "0 grams." I would always get a Coke with my fast food (take the "s" out of "fast" and see what you get) and most often I would say "no ice" so I could get the full 20 ounce serving of pure sugarfied delicious Coke. Convinced that there was sugar in Coke, I called the Coke headquarters in Atlanta. I asked how many grams of sugar are in one can of Coke.

"It's right here on our website sir," the customer service agent said. "There are 27 grams of sugar in one serving of Coke, it's listed under carbohydrates."

*Sneaky, sneaky!*

Sugar technically is a form of carbohydrate. But what was most shocking is that the agent said one serving is "8 ounces." Who goes out and buys an 8-ounce serving of Coke? No one! It's not sold in that amount. So in one 16-ounce bottle of Coke I was getting 54 grams of sugar.

Do that twice in a day and your body's immune system is likely to be 33% less effective. Through high fructose corn syrup and soda alone my body was easily getting over 220 grams of diabetes causing, fat producing sugar, each day. All of that sugar is converted to calories to be used as energy. What we don't burn off as energy the body will conveniently store as fat in unwanted places throughout our bodies. And with all of that excess sugar in my system my body conveniently and regularly began to store that sugar as fat over the last 20 years. It was more than I needed and I wasn't exercising.

There were some things I ate that I knew were loaded with sugar. There were many other things I consumed that I had no idea was sugar-rich because the sugar was hidden in high fructose corn syrup (HFCS). Since the 1990s, virtually all non-diet soft drinks— including most popular fruit juices and sports drinks— have been sweetened with high–fructose corn syrup (HFCS). Corn sweeteners, primarily HFCS, have eclipsed regular sugar as the ingredient of choice for beverage and food manufacturers, with the exception of some few microbrewed sodas. I got most of my excess sugar from high fructose corn syrup that was used in products in great amounts, unbeknownst to me. One of my personal commitments to become more informed was to read, read again, and then re-read all food labels!

When reading a food's listed ingredients, its largest quantity is listed first, the second largest listed next and so on. High fructose corn syrup is just as sweet as sugar, but less expensive than sugar. HFCS boosts America's farming industry significantly as was intended when it first hit shelves through cereal products back in the 1960s. Whereas natural sugars that you find in an apple, per se, will naturally produce two chemicals that solely reduce your appetite, high fructose corn syrup doesn't produce those chemicals. You can eat a bowl of breakfast cereal covered with HFCS and be just as hungry when you are done as you were before you started eating.

By reading labels, I found out HFCS was in everything! My sports drink, ketchup (almost one third sugar), bread, bar-b-que sauce, my sodas, punch, sweet teas, syrup, all of my favorite sweet snacks, and the list goes on and on. I decided if I am in the store and I picked up a food product that listed HFCS first, second, or third in the ingredients listing, I would pretend it actually said "poison." According to the book *Sugar Busters*, the rate of the diagnosis of diabetes in America from the 1950s until now parallels the rate of America's consumption of refined sugar in its diet.

The second food I targeted for elimination was potato products. I had no idea that potatoes were served with virtually every meal in America until the six weeks I went cold turkey. They are served scalloped, mashed, baked, French-fried, waffle fried, seasoned fried, etc. When I ate out, which is often because I travel so frequently, I had to regularly ask for the potato product served with my meal to be replaced by vegetables. Some experts say French Fries (starch) for example are worse and convert to higher glycemic levels than pure sugar. Hear me when I say: Your body WAS NOT MADE TO

HANDLE THOSE LEVELS OF BLOOD SUGAR PEAKS!

I feel sorry for the old Steve who used to ensure potatoes were being served with his meals and would even ask for a super size to help fill him up. That old Steve didn't know it was a suicidal request. All of those carbohydrates were being converted to sugars. Since he was not exercising, the calories that were not being burned as energy were being stored as fat throughout his body. The same is the case with pasta and white bread… carbs, carbs, carbs! When it comes to pasta some consider it not so much a sugar threat because its glycemic index is lower than table sugar, white bread, and white rice. The glycemic index, glycaemic index, or GI is a measure of the effects of carbohydrates on blood sugar levels.

Carbohydrates that break down quickly during digestion and release glucose rapidly into the bloodstream have a high GI. Carbohydrates that break down more slowly, releasing glucose more gradually into the bloodstream, have a low GI. In reality though, many use pasta as a carbohydrate rich food used to pack on the pounds. Pasta has a high calorie density. An average serving can have as many as 800-1000 calories. It's a great complex carbohydrate if you are trying to gain weight.

White sugar and white bread are in the same category as pasta—calorie dense foods. The only difference being they have very weak nutritional value. The debate continues over the benefits of enriched white bread versus 100% whole wheat bread. Whenever you

read that something has been 'enriched' it means that so
much of the good stuff was lost through the refining
process they had to put stuff into it to make it better for
you.

"Enriched flour is absorbed by the body not
as wheat or a grain, in which case your body could
use the energy slowly and effectively, but as a
starch. That is because the wheat germ has been
stripped from the flour; the FDA specifically states
that enriched flour cannot have greater than 5
percent wheat germ. Okay, so this stuff has been
stripped down and you're left with a starch (that
makes a nice paste when combined with water).
How does your body react to pure starch? The same
way it reacts to pure sugar! The consumption of
enriched white flour or a product containing
enriched white flour causes your body to scream
through the ride on a sugar high/low roller coaster.

Enriched white flour also makes people fatter.
White flour is really nothing more than refined
carbohydrates. According to a study that was
referenced by Natural News, Americans are eating
enough extra calories (mostly through refined
carbs) to add three pounds of body fat per month to
their weight. Carbs should come from unrefined
sources, like fresh organic fruits and vegetables.

Not from something that's been processed
and bleached and then had trace amounts of
synthetic nutrients added back in so that the
'industry' can sleep at night." – Dr. Edward Group[1]

# Chapter 3

# Something Ain't Right

When your glucose level is excessively high, your body has a hard time processing sugar. Your mouth gets dry which causes thirst, which is then followed by your attempt to satisfy that thirst. When you satisfy that thirst, you know what comes next... the bathroom.

In February of 2005, I was in New Jersey doing a series of talks when it hit me... uncontrollable thirst. Wow, was I thirsty. Sitting in the Diner, having lunch that day, I didn't know my blood sugar was in the stroke zone. The very thing that was making me thirsty was the very thing I was consuming—sugar. In one sitting I drank eight 20-ounce refills of raspberry sweet tea loaded with sugar. I then ran to the bathroom several times. By the time that we got back on the road for our afternoon assemblies, my vision was too blurred to see the expressway signs overhead. That scared me. I called my wife, a health care professional, and relayed to her my symptoms.

"Sounds like type-2 diabetes," she said.

I had never heard of type-2 diabetes. When I was growing up the adults talked about somebody having "sugar." They never called it diabetes type 1 or 2. A part of me wishes that they did, at least I would have had a familiarity with the disease. Once we arrived at the school, my mouth was so dry I had to present my talk with a bottle of water in my hand to lubricate my mouth to form words every few phrases. Twenty minutes into a forty-minute presentation I had to go to the bathroom.

*"Something ain't right,"* I said to myself.

After returning to Washington, DC I went to the doctor. He was alarmed. It was my first diagnosis of a high sugar level. He prescribed medication and restricted my diet. After several months I was back to normal. After some brief research I discovered I have a high predisposition for diabetes. My father is a diabetic. His sister died from complications of her diabetes. His brother died from complications of his diabetes. And as my doctor put it, my father gave me a gift that causes my insulin production to be sluggish; which means that I have to take extra precautions not to become a victim of diabetes.

This all happened in the year 2005. That incident gave me a heightened awareness of the disease but did not prompt me to lose weight. It wasn't until August of 2007 that I got serious. I began to notice more and more individuals who suffered from complications of diabetes. I was stunned to find out that one of my NFL heroes, Jack Tatum, the retired hard hitting free safety of the Oakland Raiders, suffered from diabetes and had several toes and part of his leg removed before dying from a massive heart attack.

Ron Springs, the famous Dallas Cowboy running back, developed type-2 diabetes. He eventually had to have his right foot amputated and then he experienced kidney failure. He was put on a transplant list because none of his family members were a match for a kidney transplant. His former teammate Everson Walls, a match, donated his kidney for the transplant and it saved Springs' life. Eight months later he went into the hospital for what was supposed to be minor surgery. He never recovered, went into a coma that left him permanently incapacitated mentally and physically.

This thing is serious. Below is a list of complications resulting from diabetes.

- Bladder Control Problems
- Diabetes, Heart Disease, and Stroke
- Diabetic Neuropathies: Foot and leg pain from the Nerve Damage
- Diabetic Retinopathy (Eye Disease) loss of sight
- Erectile Dysfunction
- Erection Problems
-  Hypoglycemia (Low Blood Glucose)
- Kidney Disease of Diabetes
- Kidney Failure
- Sexual and Urologic Problems
- Stomach Nerve Damage (Gastro paresis)

"Over 2.2 million African Americans have diabetes; 1.5 million have been diagnosed and 730,000 have not yet been diagnosed. There are 4 times as many African Americans diagnosed with diabetes today as there were in 1968. For every 6 white Americans who have diabetes, 10 African

Americans have the disease. Among African Americans 20 years and older, the prevalence of diabetes is 8.2 percent compared with 4.8 percent among non-Latino whites.

Death rates for people with diabetes are 27 percent higher for blacks compared with whites. Diabetes is the fifth leading cause of death for those ages 45 years or older. One of the problems for African Americans with diabetes is that they are more likely to develop diabetes complications and experience greater disability from the complications than whites. The frequency of diabetic retinopathy (vision impairment) is 40 to 50 percent higher in African Americans than in white Americans.

African Americans with diabetes experience kidney failure (also called 'end-stage renal disease') about four times more often than diabetic white Americans. In 1995, there were 27,258 new cases of kidney failure attributed to diabetes in black Americans. African Americans are much more likely to undergo a lower-extremity amputation than white or Latinos with diabetes. In 1994, there were 13,000 amputations among black people with diabetes, involving 155,000 days in the hospital."[2]

Recently we contacted a former employee to come back to our youth center for six weeks of seasonal work. She was available to work, but unfortunately she couldn't see. For years she struggled with her diabetes. "Linda" had gone completely blind.

I owed it to myself to educate myself on issues of health and the heart. And so do you! There once was a time one would have to sit in the library for hours looking up resources, many of which were not available or were outdated, in order to learn information in a particular field of interest. Today, within a few clicks of a computer's mouse, volumes of current, specific and expert data and analysis can be right in front of you. I dedicated time regularly to study things important to weight loss that I previously had only a cursory knowledge about like metabolism, calories, high fructose corn syrup, water, etc. Becoming a student of my body made my health more than just a blip on my radar screen, but a necessary everyday "beacon of light" influence on every physical activity and everything I ate or drank. I'm not going to force you to trudge through pages of mundane facts about the aforementioned topics, but I will highlight some basic information important for the layman to know.

When it comes to weight loss, there is always a discussion on metabolism. Metabolism is the process by which your body converts what you eat and drink into energy. During this complex biochemical process, calories in food and beverages are combined with oxygen to release the energy your body needs to function. Even when you're at rest, your body needs energy for all its hidden functions such as breathing, circulating blood, adjusting hormone levels, and growing and repairing cells. People are quick to blame their metabolism for their weight gain. While it's true that metabolism is linked to weight, it may not be in the way you expect. In fact, contrary to common belief, a slow metabolism is rarely the cause of excess weight gain. Although your metabolism influences your body's basic energy needs, it's your food and beverage intake and your physical activity (or lack of it) that ultimately determines how much you weigh.

The number of calories your body uses to carry out basic functions is known as your basal metabolic rate (BMR)—what we call metabolism. Several factors determine your individual basal metabolic rate:

- Your body size and composition. The bodies of people who are larger or have more muscle burn up more calories, even at rest.
- Your sex. Men usually have less body fat and more muscle than do women of the same age and weight, making men burn more calories.
- Your age. As you get older, the amount of muscle tends to decrease and fat accounts for more of your weight, which slows down calorie burning.

Energy needs for your body's basic functions stay fairly consistent and aren't easily changed. Your basal metabolic rate accounts for about 60 to 75 percent of the calories you burn every day.

In addition to your basal metabolic rate, two other factors determine how many calories your body burns each day:

- Food processing (thermogenesis). Digesting, absorbing, transporting and storing the food you consume also takes calories. This accounts for about 10 percent of the calories used each day. For the most part, your body's energy requirement to process food stays relatively steady and isn't easily changed.

- Physical activity. Physical activity and exercise — such as playing tennis, walking to the store, chasing after the dog and any other movement — account for the rest of the calories your body burns up each day.

Your metabolism cleverly adjusts management of your body's energy according to the reserves on hand. If you don't eat breakfast, you slow down your metabolism and send the body into "hoard mode," thinking it's starving because you've gone a long period of time (frequently 8 to 10 hours or more) without food.

The management process then is to burn fewer calories and store more calories as fat. Dropping your calorie intake below 1,000 calories a day will signal to your body that you are in starvation mode, and will also slow down your metabolism. The solution is eat smaller meals more frequently. Smaller, more frequent meals keeps your blood sugar stable and provides a steady source of energy to fuel metabolism. One of the changes I made was to eat frequent meals. Every two and a half to three hours I was eating something; a meal or a snack.

In addition to eating smaller, more frequent meals, you must get enough aerobic exercise. As much as you can do is really a big help for your metabolism, and if you do exercise in the morning, you'll raise your metabolism all day.

You also should build more muscle with weight training or resistance exercise. At least two to three times a week, you should add weight training or progressive resistance exercise that builds muscle. Muscle burns more calories than fat, and the more muscle you have, the more calories you burn, even at rest!

There is never a better time to take your health more seriously. It should start today. Make a plan and stick to it. That which you persist at doing becomes easier. Not necessarily the task itself, but your ability to do the task increases. So stick to it! Activate and boost your metabolism. Change your diet. Start exercising and leave the fa(s)t foods alone!

# Chapter 4
# The Motivation

50/5

One warm summer day I came home early from work, exhausted. I was up late the night before and was on the go all day from early morning until I was able to get home that afternoon. Too tired to climb the stairs to my bedroom, I dropped my briefcase at the door, grabbed a pillow from the couch, and stretched out on my living room floor. Within a few minutes, lying comfortably snug on the carpet, I was fast asleep and home alone. It was a sound afternoon nap.

When I awoke, without thinking about it, I crawled on my hands and knees over to the couch. With a grunt and groan I used the couch to help myself get to my feet. Then it dawned on me. I was 45 years old, almost 300 pounds, but could not under my own power get up from the floor without help. I needed assistance from the couch.

My reflections and embarrassment continued. "Here I am, a former professional athlete, struggling to merely stand to my feet. How will I ever be able to bounce my future grandchildren on my knee one day or play with them on the floor? Worse yet, what if all they know about their grandpa are the stories told about him, and the pictures and videos they see, because grandpa died of a heart attack before they were born?"

My children deserve to have their father around as they negotiate the challenges of adulthood. My children need a dad who can be an active grandfather in the lives of their children one day. I owed it to my loved ones to make a commitment to be healthy! Motivation!

As a motivational speaker I've spoken to a wide variety of audiences with tips for success and strategies to excel. In the corporate world my most popular talk is, "Super Bowl Lessons From A Championship Season." I caught a glimpse of a man in the middle of one of those corporate talks in Northern Virginia. I was in a room full of marketing executives extolling the virtues of goal-setting and discipline when out of the corner of my eye I caught the reflection in the glass window of an overweight gentleman, sweating profusely, struggling to look comfortable in a "tight around the collar" suit... it was me. What a profound discredit to the wisdom I attempted to put forth. How can I authentically motivate and encourage others to greatness while I personally lived in such physical defeat? I found myself a public success but a private failure.

Not long after that I hosted an event with one of my mentors, a professional speaker named Les Brown. Another mentor and professional speaker, Willie Jolley heard that Les was in town and stopped by the event. Two of the world's renowned speakers in one place, I had to have a photo. When the professional photograph of me, Willie Jolley, and Les Brown was delivered to my office that week there was one glaring aspect of the photo that I simply couldn't overlook. They looked like the message they preached; I looked fat, out of shape and out of control. I had to do something! I had to get serious. It was not only for my health but also for the strength of my message.

The same is true for those who profess the victory of their faith on Sunday mornings but live in bondage to their dinner table at night. Mike Murdock, better known as the wisdom teacher, said we all need to walk or run a mile a day for two reasons. The first reason is that exercising will make us live longer. The second reason, he said, and this is what really got me, "some of us need to prove to God that we are not lazy." Let's face it: The reason I didn't exercise (even though I had a treadmill in my basement) was because there were times that I was simply too lazy to do so. I had healthy feet, healthy legs, and a capable body so I had to tell myself, "EXERCISE!"

Another major motivation was the result of a movie I noticed while browsing through the video store one day. Always on the go, busy, overbooked, and too often unfocused, I rarely planned my meals. I always ended up so hungry that I had to have something good, fast. McDonald's was my poison of choice. When I am "starving" I can hit the drive-thru and in minutes, inexpensively, I could have a Big Mac, those delicious Mickey D's fries, *mmmm*, and a huge cold Coke to chase it… HEAVEN! If it were breakfast, I'd get the sausage Mcgriddle (420 calories) with cinnamon melts (460 calories) and a large orange juice (20 ounces= 250 calories).

Then I rented this movie: *Super Size Me!*

While examining the influence of the fast food industry, Morgan Spurlock (writer, director, and star) personally explores the consequences on his health of a diet of solely McDonald's food for one month. Several legal suits have been brought against McDonald's restaurants with claimants stating McDonald's knowingly sells food that is unhealthy. Some of the court decisions have stated that the plaintiffs would have a claim if they could prove that eating the food every day for every meal is dangerous. As such, documentarian Morgan Spurlock conducted an unscientific experiment using himself as the guinea pig. The rules of engagement were that he ate only McDonald's for thirty days, three meals a day. If the clerk asked him if he would like the meal super sized, he had to say yes. And by the end of the thirty days, he had to have eaten every single menu item at least once.

Before starting the experiment, he was tested by three doctors: a general practitioner, a cardiologist and a gastroenterologist. All three pronounced his general health to be outstanding. They monitored him over the thirty days to ensure that he is not placing his health into irreparable damage. As a result, the then 32-year-old Spurlock gained 24½ pounds, a 13% body mass increase, developed a cholesterol level of 230 (less than 150 is normal), and experienced mood swings, sexual dysfunction, and fat accumulation to his liver that almost killed him. It took Spurlock fourteen months to lose the weight gained from his experiment.

There is too much good information in the movie to

give it a complete review here. I encourage you to download the movie for free at freedocumentaries.org. I would like to note what impacted me most.

One scene detailed the expanding waistline of Americans using random shots of busy people downtown in a busy city. Images of overweight people from all walks of life coupled with the devastating voice over of data on the declining health status of the average American and the rising population of obese Americans was simply numbing. The final shot in this scene was a rearview close up of a group of people from their shoulders to their knees with the emphasis on their midsection. They were all obese. You saw the rolls of fat, the love handles, the spare tires; everything. As the camera completed its pan from left to right it slowly began to zoom out. They were all standing in line at a McDonald's. In my mind's eye I saw myself in the line. As a McDonald's fan this movie first blew my mind, then changed my life.

One of my greatest motivations is directly tied to my mission and purpose in life. To do anything worth doing there must be enthusiasm and passion to go with purpose. One of my mentors made a profound statement one day when he identified one's greatest resource when it comes to communicating truth for life-change.

"It doesn't matter how powerful your sermon or the message you have to tell, without you the story can never be told," Myles Munroe once said.

If my health is in disrepair I cannot produce a message, no matter how insightful my message may be.

I am bound to protect my health. All that I have to say as a motivational speaker is predicated upon the strength of my physical ability to communicate my thoughts and message.

# Chapter 5
# My Secret Strategy

50/5

When it comes to basic weight loss, the body must burn more calories than it consumes. That can be done one of two ways; either consume fewer calories than normal or burn more calories than normal. In my determination to lose weight and lose it expeditiously I decided to both consume fewer calories *and* burn more calories.

As this book title indicates, I lost 50 pounds in five seconds. I have already explained my modified diet. I have never been one who found calorie counting interesting. Even today people ask me about how many calories I target to consume in a day and I have difficultly exacting my calorie intake. Fortunately an i-phone application came out that lists every restaurant, and every menu item and the calorie content of each item on the menu. I thought it would be a great idea to research my typical day and my typical meals and log the corresponding calorie data. I read that 2400 to 2600 calories a day (give or take 500) would be a good, yet challenging, range for someone in my demographic to shoot for.

My day usually began with an early stop at Starbucks for a caramel macchiato and a bran muffin.

Using Starbucks as an impromptu office, I would usually make a few phone calls after a brief reading of my inspirational thoughts for the day, then return or send a few e-mails. By 11:00 a.m. I was in the drive-thru line at McDonald's for a double cheeseburger meal, hold the ice in the Coke so I can get more Coke. I'd add a Filet-O-Fish sandwich when I was really hungry. If my day got too busy I could have the same meal by 2:30 or 3:00 p.m. By 6:00 I was having dinner at my youth center with my students. At 7:30 p.m. I was stopping at 7-Eleven on my way home to pick up a Hostess yellow cupcake and 16 ounce bottle of Nestlé's strawberry milk. Upon arriving at home I'd eat dinner with my family and before the night was out I'd be snacking on two peanut butter and jelly sandwiches. Can somebody say, "SUICIDE!"

I was killing myself and didn't even know it. Remember my calorie goal was 2600 per day tops. My calorie intake for the typical day excluding dinner was as follows:

| | |
|---|---|
| Caramel Macchiato (Grande) | 270 Calories |
| Bran Muffin | 420 Calories |
| Double Cheeseburger | 490 Calories |
| Large French Fries | 380 Calories |
| Filet-O-Fish Sandwich | 470 Calories |
| Medium Coke | 210 Calories |
| Hostess Cupcake | 175 Calories |
| Nestlé's Strawberry Milk | 230 Calories |
| (2) Peanut butter and Jelly | 600 Calories |

Excluding dinner at the youth center and dinner at home with my family I was consuming 3,245 calories. Remember, some days I'd make two trips to McDonald's. That's another 1,550 calories. If we add in the average dinner, which can be anywhere from 600-1000 calories, I was averaging about 5,000-7,000 calories a day with zero exercising. At 45 years old I was a walking heart attack, stroke or health emergency waiting to happen.

Cutting calories, that's the easy part. All it takes is a little planning and a little determination. Mix in a large helping of self-discipline and the calorie intake will drop. Now *burning* calories, most would consider to be the hard part. With a little creativity, time, and opportunity, I was able to make burning calories almost second nature. I imagined that calories were all around me and all I had to do was discover them and burn them. For example, I treated escalators, moving sidewalks in airports, and elevators (up to three floors) all to be health hazards. I would walk or take the stairs instead. Being in and out of airports because of the demand of my work I could easily burn calories with a brisk walk to my gate without the use of a moving sidewalk or tram as I carried my briefcase and carry-on bag.

I especially remember being in the Atlanta airport where they post the distance between terminals. It's almost 1500 meters from the first concourse to the last. With briefcase in hand and my bag hanging from my shoulder, a swift walk topped off by a steady climb of three flights of stairs gave me an incredible burn and the elimination of dozens of calories.

Watching television became a workout. Commercials gave me a chance to do push-ups in sets of ten. Through a half hour television show I could easily complete over 100 push-ups. You might think that 100 push-ups a day is not much. But they activate the large pectoral muscles. Toned muscles feast on calories even at rest. So I may have only done 100 push-ups over a 30-minute period, but long after the push-ups are done, the "pecs" are still burning calories. Muscle is much more active than fat. That's one reason why the experts recommend weight training to reduce fat. The proper routine will not give you thickness and mass but rather definition and toning. Toned muscles are your allies in burning calories. The hungriest muscles are your largest. Your largest muscles are between your waist and knees. These muscles are your quadriceps, hamstrings, and gluteus maximus.

If you can't make it to the gym, I guarantee that if you do freestanding squats without weight at the rate of 3 sets of 15-20, 3 days a week, you will gradually see weight reduction. Once those big body muscles start exercising on a regular basis, you are destined to enter the fat burning zone.

I stopped trying to find the closest parking space at the mall and grocery store and instead intentionally park far away. *Why?* Because I'm always looking for calories to burn. I stopped sending my children up and down the stairs at home to get "things" for me and I started getting them myself, even if I just climbed those stairs and have to go back up because somewhere in my affliction of adult attention deficit disorder I forgot what I went upstairs to get.

The calories are all around us; let's find them and burn them. On vacation for example, I volunteered to carry my great-niece who was 3-years old at the time, on my shoulders while we hiked. *Why?* Calories. Sometimes I didn't feel like running my two-mile route so I grabbed my headset and ipod and walked a mile and a half anyway. *Why?* Calories! Calories! Calories!

When I was obese I did zero exercising. And even today, the thirty-minute walk I take is lightyears better than doing nothing. I must be determined to be healthy. Men particular to my demographic (middle-aged, African American, with a diabetic heritage) are falling prey at alarming rates to diabetes, heart disease, stroke, and other "dis-case."

As Dr. Dobson once said on his *Focus On The Family* radio program shortly after he recovered from a heart attack, "When you are lying on your back in the hospital with tubes in every hole in your face, 30-minutes a day, three times a week seems like nothing!"

The following 3 pages give you some guidelines for approximately how many calories you can burn doing a wide variety of activites.

## One Hour Activity

| Cardio Activity | 155 lbs. | 190 lbs. |
| --- | --- | --- |
| Running, 12 minute mile pace | 562 | 689 |
| Running, 10 minute mile pace | 703 | 862 |
| Running, 8 minute mile pace | 879 | 1,077 |
| Running, 7 minute mile pace | 984 | 1,207 |
| Running up stairs | 1,055 | 1,293 |
| Freestyle lap swimming with vigorous effort | 703 | 862 |
| Freestyle lap swimming with moderate effort | 562 | 689 |
| Bicycling, moderate effort | 562 | 689 |
| Bicycling, very fast | 844 | 1,034 |
| Mountain biking | 598 | 733 |
| Stationary bicycling, moderate | 492 | 603 |
| Stationary bicycling, vigorous | 738 | 905 |
| Walking, pushing or pulling stroller | 176 | 215 |
| Walking up stairs | 562 | 689 |
| Walking 3 mph, level surface | 245 | 302 |
| Walking 4.5 mph level surface | 316 | 388 |
| Walking 3.5 mph uphill | 422 | 517 |
| Stationary rowing, moderate effort | 492 | 603 |
| Stationary rowing, vigorous effort | 598 | 733 |

## Resistance Training

| | 155 lbs. | 190 lbs. |
| --- | --- | --- |
| Weightlifting, vigorous effort | 422 | 517 |
| Weightlifting, light/moderate | 211 | 259 |

## Recreation

| | 155 lbs. | 190 lbs. |
| --- | --- | --- |
| Stream fishing in waders | 422 | 517 |
| Ice fishing, sitting | 141 | 172 |

## Winter Sports

| | 155 lbs. | 190 lbs. |
| --- | --- | --- |
| Ice hockey | 562 | 689 |
| Ice skating, 9 mph | 387 | 474 |
| Ice skating, over 9 mph | 633 | 776 |

| Winter Sports (continued) | 155 lbs. | 190 lbs. |
| --- | --- | --- |
| Cross-country skiing, 4-4.9 mph | 562 | 689 |
| Cross-country skiing, 5-7.9 mph | 633 | 776 |
| Cross-country skiing, uphill | 1,160 | 1,422 |
| Curling | 281 | 345 |
| Downhill skiing, moderate effort | 422 | 517 |
| Sledding, tobogganing, bobsledding, luge | 492 | 603 |

## Chores

| | 155 lbs. | 190 lbs. |
| --- | --- | --- |
| Washing car, vigorous effort | 316 | 388 |
| Vacuuming | 176 | 215 |
| Grocery shopping | 246 | 302 |
| Making your bed | 141 | 172 |
| Moving furniture | 422 | 517 |
| Sweeping | 281 | 345 |
| Auto repair | 211 | 259 |
| Installing rain gutters | 422 | 517 |
| Hanging storm windows | 352 | 431 |
| Painting | 316 | 388 |
| Chopping wood | 422 | 517 |
| Mowing the lawn | 422 | 517 |
| Operating a snowblower | 316 | 388 |
| Shoveling snow | 422 | 517 |
| Bailing hay | 562 | 689 |
| Milking a cow | 211 | 259 |

## Sports

| | 155 lbs. | 190 lbs. |
| --- | --- | --- |
| Basketball | 562 | 689 |
| Billiards | 176 | 215 |
| Bowling | 211 | 259 |
| Boxing, punching a heavy bag | 422 | 517 |
| Football, touch or flag | 562 | 689 |
| Golf, carrying clubs | 387 | 474 |
| Golf, using a cart | 246 | 302 |
| Handball | 844 | 1,034 |
| Judo, jujitsu, karate, kickboxing, tae kwon do | 703 | 862 |

## Sports (continued)

| | | |
|---|---|---|
| Racquetball | 492 | 603 |
| Rope jumping, moderate effort | 703 | 862 |
| Soccer | 492 | 603 |
| Tai chi | 281 | 345 |
| Tennis, singles | 562 | 689 |
| Backpacking | 492 | 603 |
| Hiking | 422 | 517 |
| Kayaking | 352 | 431 |
| Snorkeling | 352 | 431 |
| Surfing, body or board | 211 | 259 |

## At Work

| | | |
|---|---|---|
| Desk work | 127 | 155 |
| Carpentry | 246 | 302 |
| Fire fighting, climbing ladder with full gear | 773 | 948 |
| Policing, making an arrest | 562 | 689 |
| Sitting in a meeting | 105 | 129 |
| Bartending | 176 | 215 |
| Making photocopies | 176 | 215 |
| Walking around the office at a moderate pace | 246 | 302 |

# Chapter 6

50/5

# You Are Not Sick, You Are Thirsty!

Every team I've ever been on has always insisted on each player drinking enough water. Consequently throughout my life, I have had a heightened sensitivity to the value and the need for athletes to be hydrated. At times I have taken for granted my body's need for water. Outside of competition, there were many times that I did not prioritize my suggested daily intake of water. However, as a result of my research for improving my health, I finally discovered aspects of water and hydration that gave the role of water in my life tremendous significance. Water isn't part of the solution; it is the core of the solution. Of all the vitamins, supplements, and nutrients that our organs need to survive, water is the body's freeway to distribute vitamins, supplements, nutrients, and energy to those organs.

Probably the single most important change I made in my diet was my water consumption. I established water as my primary refreshment for each meal. Too many of us are drinking most of our calories instead through unhealthy drinks. I began keeping a bottle of water with me in the car. Between meals I would sip on water and snack on almonds to keep myself from entering the "Red Zone." The Red Zone is that point where I feel like I'm starving and I have to satisfy my hunger quickly and inexpensively. That's a very dangerous place for me to be. Water helps me avoid that place. After a while, drinking lots of water every day got boring. While watching a health and fitness program, the expert suggested to "make your water sexy" when you get bored of drinking water.

"Add some lemon, ice, or carbonation to your water," she said. That's what I did. I can't explain why carbonated water became my drink of choice. I can tell you that I can drink carbonated water with just a splash of lemon all day.

I picked up a used copy of a highly recommended book by F. Batmanghelidj, M.D. entitled *Your Body's Many Cries For Water*. In it I uncovered a wealth of knowledge about water and my body. The subtitle is: *You're Not Sick, You're Thirsty*. Water is the secret cure to most things that ail us. Most of us confuse hunger with thirst. Our reaction to the notion of hunger is to eat, when often times we are actually thirsty.

There once was a time when I'd go to a restaurant and have three Cokes while waiting on my food. Today I simply ask for a pitcher of water. By the time my food arrives I will have had at least two waters and the edge of my hunger has been eased. Additionally from that same book I learned about how critical water is to the rebuilding process of the body's cell structure. I had no idea that every night each cell in our body puts on a "hardhat" and begins the nightly construction work of regeneration. Chronic lack of sleep, or poor-quality sleep, has an incredibly negative effect on the way we feel and on the way we look. When we are asleep, our cells rebuild and repair themselves (the growth hormone functions only at night). If you don't sleep, this function is impaired. That's why it's important for us to get a good night's sleep. Some experts say men need fewer hours of sleep each night than women (someone may joke that's because women do more work).

The reality is men and women both need about 7.5 to 8.5 hours of sleep a night. The cells need quality time to rebuild and regenerate. A special paste called H20–water–holds each cell together. The male body is made up of about 60% water, the female 55%. Our whole existence is dependent on water, yet we too often take it for granted.

Decide today to start your mornings right: Morning is when you are most full of toxins and dehydrated. Every morning I start my day with a big glass of water and I proclaim aloud, "This is the most important glass of water I will drink all day!" Reach for a big glass of water first thing in the morning–even before coffee. This water in the morning really gets the blood flowing.

- Drink a glass of water when you get up and another when you go to bed.
- Take regular water breaks.
- Avoid relying on sodas to provide your fluid needs.

- Drink water before and after food; ideally drink a glass of water half an hour before you eat your meal and half an hour after the meal.

You can drink water with meals, and drink water anytime your body feels like it. You should always drink water both prior to eating and after eating to support the digestive process. The stomach depends on water to help digest food, and lack of water makes it harder for nutrients to be broken down and used as energy. The liver, which dictates where all nutrients go, also needs water to help convert stored fat into usable energy. If you are dehydrated, the kidneys turn to the liver for backup, diminishing the liver's ability to metabolize stored fat. The resulting reduced blood volume will interfere with your body's ability to remove toxins and supply your cells with adequate nutrients.

Keep a water bottle by your side at all the times. Use either bottled water or tap water, and carry it with you everywhere, to the gym, in your car, to your office. Start by adding water to your daily regiment during the first week of exercise, and then incorporate more as needed. The point is not to wait until you're thirsty to drink.

Keep water flowing before, during, and after workouts. Don't forget to balance your water intake with sodium intake. Drink at least 1 liter of water for every 60 minutes of exercise. Drink more if it's hot. During exercise, such as playing a sport on a hot summer day, you can lose up to 2 liters per hour of fluid per hour. Water and a balanced salt is your best bet to keep healthy and hydrated. During exercise, it is recommended to replenish fluid at least every 20 minutes.

Dr. Batmanghelidj, in *Your Body's Many Cries for Water*, was able to trace 37 known diseases and ailments back to dehydration. I became a water freak. My complexion became clearer, skin healthier, and energy higher all because I took water seriously. When I was uninformed I use to think since Kool-Aid, soda, sweet teas, and sweet drinks were made with water then there must be some benefit in drinking them. Because those drinks are loaded with so many unhealthy ingredients, the work the body has to do to extract the good from the bad stresses the liver too much rather than getting the pure natural benefit of a cool glass of water. Refer to the chart on the next page for a list of the common benefits of water to your body.

# 10 Benefits of Drinking Water

1. Water is absolutely essential to the human body's survival. A person can live for about a month without food, but only about a week without water.
2. Water helps to maintain healthy body weight by increasing metabolism and regulating appetite.
3. Water leads to increased energy levels. The most common cause of daytime fatigue is actually mild dehydration.
4. Drinking adequate amounts of water can decrease the risk of certain types of cancers, including colon cancer, bladder cancer, and breast cancer.
5. For a majority of sufferers, drinking water can significantly reduce joint and/or back pain.
6. Water leads to overall greater health by flushing out wastes and bacteria that can cause disease.
7. Water can prevent and alleviate headaches.
8. Water naturally moisturizes skin and ensures proper cellular formation underneath layers of skin to give it a healthy, glowing appearance.
9. Water aids in the digestion process and prevents constipation.
10. Water is the primary mode of transportation for all nutrients in the body and is essential for proper circulation.

# Chapter 7
# The Bonus Burn

**50/5**

As I mentioned earlier you lose weight when you burn more calories than you consume. I am a firm believer that one of the most effective ways to safely burn calories is to run or jog. There are a variety of ways to accomplish your cardio goals of weight loss. Cardio is really a modern term that has grown to replace aerobic exercise. To avoid the stigma of the aerobic craze of the 70s, people switched to using the word *cardio* when discussing it relative to fitness and strength training programs to disassociate with the aerobics-only phenomenon. What I call the "bonus burn" is to couple my cardio activity with resistance or weight training.

When people think about weight training they often become intimidated by the idea of hitting the gym and being stared down by muscle bound "Hulks" that are smirking at your flabby arms, un-toned butt, and pudgy midsection. Remember it's not about other people and their impressions of you, but rather you and your commitment to live! So whether you have access to a gym, weight training facility, weights at home or not, there are some great benefits that the serious health conscious individual should be aware of and implement.

When you do resistance training (lift weights) the benefit goes far beyond your exercise. As I said, muscle is quite more active than fat. That means that after you have stimulated your muscles through resistance training, they continue to burn calories even while you are at rest. Another misnomer is that if you lift weights you will put on weight and become thick and muscular. If your routine consists of very heavy weight, few sets and few repetitions, then you are right. Your body will recruit muscle fibers that yield strength and size. However, if you lighten the load and do more sets with higher repetitions, your body will recruit muscle fibers that yield endurance and muscle definition. That's where you want to be, light weight with many repetitions. When I say light weight, I'm speaking of a weight that you can do 10-12 repetitions for 2-3 sets when you begin. After a few weeks you should be able to do the same weight 12-15 times for 2-3 sets.

"Where do I begin?" you might ask.

I'm no expert although I have been involved in weight training most of my life. I would suggest that you develop a routine. Group your weight training days by the body parts you intend to develop. I never want to be in the gym too long, so I don't try to do everything every day. I separate my days by doing my chest, shoulders, and back one day then legs and arms the next. I figure I need my arms to work my chest, shoulders and back so I exercise them separately on the days I work my legs. For each body part I do at least two exercises (three would be a plus). Your muscles need four things to adequately respond and grow; stimulus (resistance training), flexibility, nutrition, and rest. You should not do every body part every day. For some reason, the abdominals are an exception to this. Experts say you can work them every day.  Yippee!

## Good News and Bad News

The bad news is this will be challenging. In other words: there will be pain. There will be soreness the first few days, discouragement will come, and remaining consistent can become more and more of a challenge. As my coach Dan Reeves once said, "If it were easy, we'd all be champions."

The good news is the calories and subsequent fat will burn away expeditiously! Remember what Stephen Covey says in *Seven Habits of Highly Successful People*:

> "The common denominator of success is simply the fact that successful people make a habit of doing what failures don't like to do.  It's not that they enjoy doing it.  The strength of their purpose is greater than their dislike."

How bad do you want it?  Allow your passion to out-burn your pain. I am testifying to you that steady cardio exercise (running, swimming, jogging, walking, etc.)  coupled  with  basic  resistance  training  will produce a fit and healthy you. And when the fat falls, a toned and defined fit-frame will be visible.

Resistance training is a way of telling your muscles, "You all can't just hangout on my body and do nothing, you've got to help me burn away the fat."

If you do not have access to a gym, don't fret, all is not lost. The next time you are on Facebook, open a new tab and in that window do a Google search for "Resistance training without weights" and begin to document all the things you can do at home to improve your strength and tone your body. On the following page I will give you one man's synopsis of a beginner's resistance training routine. I am not going to describe what each exercise is, you can look that up on your own (Google search).

Keep in mind that the object is to use a light enough weight to get multiple sets and 10-12 repetitions each set. As Lee Haney, former Mr. Universe, would say, "Drive 55, you stay alive!" You get 20% more out our your workout by choosing a lighter weight. If your physical fitness level is such that you can't use any weight at all at first, then no weight it is! The key ingredient is consistency. If it's going to be three days a week, then let it be three days a week for six weeks, then chart your improvement. Establish a routine, and change your lifestyle!

# SAMPLE RESISTANCE TRAINING SCHEDULE

## DAY 1:

CHEST
Bench press
Incline press
Dumbbell flys

SHOULDERS
Seated behind the neck press
Light weight lateral raises

BACK
Lat pull downs
Bent rows

ABDOMINALS
Crunches
Leg raises

## DAY 2:

QUADRICEPS
Leg extensions
Lunges

HAMSTRINGS
Leg curls
Dead lifts

GLUTEUS MAXIMUS
Squats
Step ups

ABDOMINALS
Crunches
Leg raises

# Chapter 8
## Summary

50/5

50 pounds in 5 seconds! It began like that, but ended up being a total of almost 100 pounds lost over 13 months. I didn't know how far gone I was until I lost the weight. Today when I see pictures of the old Steve I feel sorry for him. I see the tiredness in his eyes, the sweat on his brow, and the struggle in his face all from his obesity. In fact, I grieve often for the people I see laboring to carry around excess tonnage.

I recently saw an old friend at a ballgame. He had gained so much weight I almost wanted to cry for him. He could barely climb the stairs of the bleachers to find his seat. What a scary way to do life, having death at your door because of your lifestyle. I grieve when I go shopping and see people waddling behind shopping carts loaded with "poisons." That was me, unaware. I am overwhelmingly aware of how serious this is. I was one of those people not many years ago. I was fortunate that I didn't have a life-threatening crisis to convince me to make a change. Even though I've made the changes, I still have to monitor my blood glucose levels. As my doctor recently told me, my father gave me a gift unintentionally: a diabetic heritage. I am constantly aware that my father is a diabetic. I am reminded again that my aunt, his sister, was a diabetic and died from complications of her struggle with the disease. And I am reminded that my uncle, his brother, a diabetic and amputee, died as a result of his diabetes. My body is sluggish in its ability to produce insulin. I must maintain my health to avoid diabetes.

As a result of dietary changes, my taste buds have adapted. There once was a time that I practically turned my coffee into hot chocolate with all of the sugar and creamer I added. Today, I can only take my coffee without sugar, and a little milk. I prefer sugar free drinks with no artificial sweeteners. The scope of this writing won't allow me to go into detail on the most popular artificial sweetener, aspartame. When you get a moment, study it on your own. The reports have convinced me to end my consumption of all diet drinks and products that use it. On occasion I'll have a drink of sweet tea made at home by one of my daughters and I cringe. Too much sugar! Never thought I'd say that. I have conditioned myself not to need desser,t but rather enjoy dessert in moderation only when I want to. Although in the beginning I went cold turkey, I eventually got to the point where I'd allow myself one or two desserts a week, tops.

In the beginning I was running at least 6 or 7 days a week. My regular run became a 3.2-mile run in downtown Washington, DC. At first I was too heavy to run and resorted to a 30 minute walk. The walk, weeks later became a jog. The jog became a run. Today I'm running 3-4 days a week or swimming 30 minutes a day. Gone are the days of not being able to talk while running. Now when my wife and I run we talk back and forth for the entire run. It's a great time of bonding. We run together and recently competed in a 5K race together. Even my stamina for presentations has increased. I no longer need a towel to wipe the sweat; sometimes I don't sweat at all. My friend put it in perspective. The 100 pounds that I carried around would be like me carrying a 45 pound weight in each hand everywhere I went. As a weightlifter I know how difficult it is simply to put a 45 pound plate on the barbell. It's hard to conceive I had been carrying around two of those plates for 20 years.

How do I keep the weight off? It was never a matter of losing weight as it was a matter of instituting a lifestyle change. I changed the way I do life. It took diet, exercise, motivation, and education. It took consistency. Now, it's simply the way I live. Because of these changes I'm doing things I haven't done in years. They may be trite to you, but they're significant to me. I can sit down, cross my legs, and wiggle my foot! I sit in the middle seat on the airplane without being "squished." I bend over and tie my shoe without sitting down or finding a pedestal to rest my foot. I can go to the restaurant and have enough food left over to take home a doggy-bag.

On any given day I can put on my running shoes and go out on a 3-mile run. I don't have to go to the big and tall store to shop for clothes. In fact, my entire wardrobe has changed. I wear colors other than black!

To top it off, I really look 10 years younger than I actually am and it feels good. There really are no shortcuts.

To be completely honest, I fell off the wagon from Thanksgiving of 2008 through New Years of 2009. I went from 215 pounds back to 245 pounds. I put the brakes on, righted the ship, and got back on the grind. If I can do it, you can do it too. Eat right and exercise and over time the changes will come. Find your motivation. Research on your own some of the information I briefly mentioned in this book. Make the tough decisions at the meal table. Each time you make a difficult decision you become stronger. The harder you run or walk today, the easier your run or walk will be tomorrow. Find a variety of ways to burn calories. You lose weight when you burn more calories than you consume. Burn those calories, consume fewer calories and watch the weight drop. Reread this book, and make notes. The small decisions you make today will add up to great gains in your life. Document your progress. Take before and after photos, and then tell your story!

Live life! Live long! Live blessed!

## Some additional Resources:

www.freedocumentaries.org
www.allaboutwater.org
www.watercure.com
www.bettersleep.org
www.womenfitness.net
www.mercola.com
www.bodybuilding.com

### Book:
*Your Body's Many Cries for Water: You Are Not Sick, You Are Thirsty* by Fereydoon Batmanghelidj. (July 1, 1995)

### Movie:
*Super Size Me*
Genre: Documentary, Special Interest
Rated: PG-13 for language, sex and drug references, and a graphic medical procedure

### References:
1 http://www.globalhealingcenter.com/natural-health/enriched-white-flour/

2 Excerpted and adapted from *Diabetes in African Americans Fact Sheet*, National Diabetes Information National Institute of Diabetes and Digestive and Kidney Diseases

# About the Author

Steve Fitzhugh is a nationally known and accomplished inspirational and motivational speaker. As a former member of the Denver Broncos of the National Football League, Steve has used his platform to reach over 1 million students in America with a message of hope, the value of good decision-making and the virtue of a committed drug-free lifestyle. Steve has successfully been able to blend his humor, experiences in the NFL, the story of his personal tragedy and his timeless antidotes of success and significance into engaging and entertaining presentations.

As an author, Steve articulately communicates through his writings with clear insights and easy to apply principles designed to help the reader become engaged in self-education and life-change. A husband, father, writer, poet, and life enthusiast, Steve has an uncommon ability to connect with both young and old with tools for personal success and professional effectiveness. Youth workers glean insights from his over 25 years of experience in work with students. Readers enjoy his writings and audiences enjoy his speaking, and the youth appreciate his ability to enter their world and spur them on to great heights and new precedents of accomplishment.

Connect with Steve: www.PowerMoves.org

www.ingramcontent.com/pod-product-compliance
Lightning Source LLC
Chambersburg PA
CBHW060521280326
41933CB00014B/3057